Juicing For Beginners

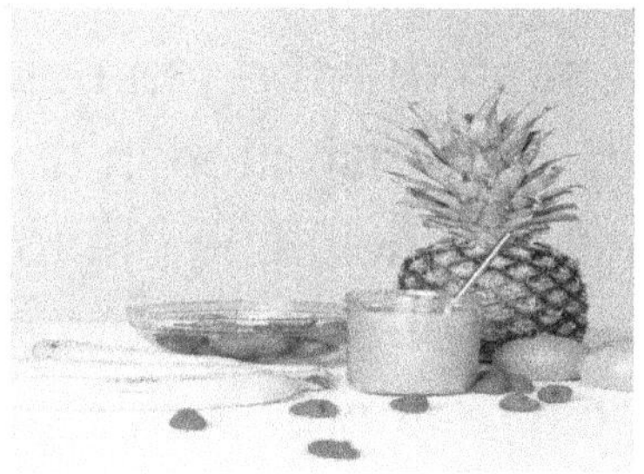

Easy and essential Juicing recipes to making healthy and detoxifying juices with troubleshooting

Megan farmer

TABLE OF CONTENT

Introduction

In a quaint town nestled between rolling hills, where the aroma of ripe orchards filled the air, lived a community seeking a path to wellness. One day, a mysterious figure arrived with crates bursting with vibrant fruits and vegetables. This enigmatic newcomer introduced the townsfolk to the art of juicing.

Intrigued by the promise of revitalization, curious minds gathered to learn the secrets of extracting liquid gold from nature's bounty. The mysterious mentor, adorned in colorful attire, revealed the transformative power of juicing for beginners. As hands eagerly gripped juicers and the hum of machinery

echoed, a journey into a healthier
lifestyle began.

The townspeople, from young adults to
wise elders, embraced the kaleidoscope
of flavors that danced on their palates.
The vibrant elixirs not only nourished
their bodies but also ignited a communal
spirit. As the sun dipped below the
horizon, laughter echoed through the
town square, and the newfound juicing
enthusiasts toasted to a brighter,
healthier tomorrow.

The mysterious figure vanished into the
night, leaving behind a legacy of
wellness that would ripple through
generations. And so, the town embarked
on a flavorful journey, guided by the
wisdom imparted by a stranger who had
gifted them the key to a vibrant life –
juicing for beginners.

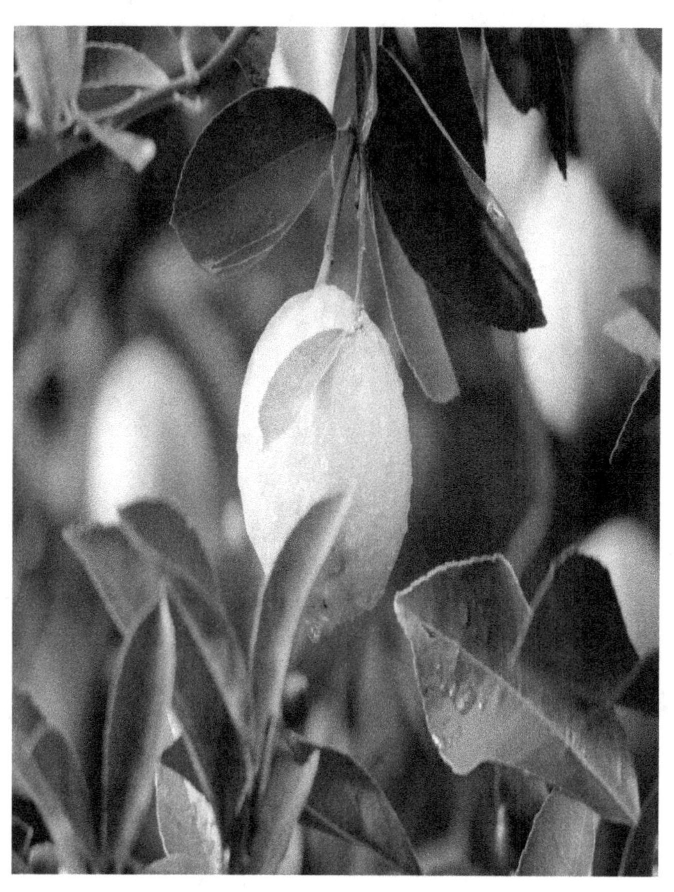

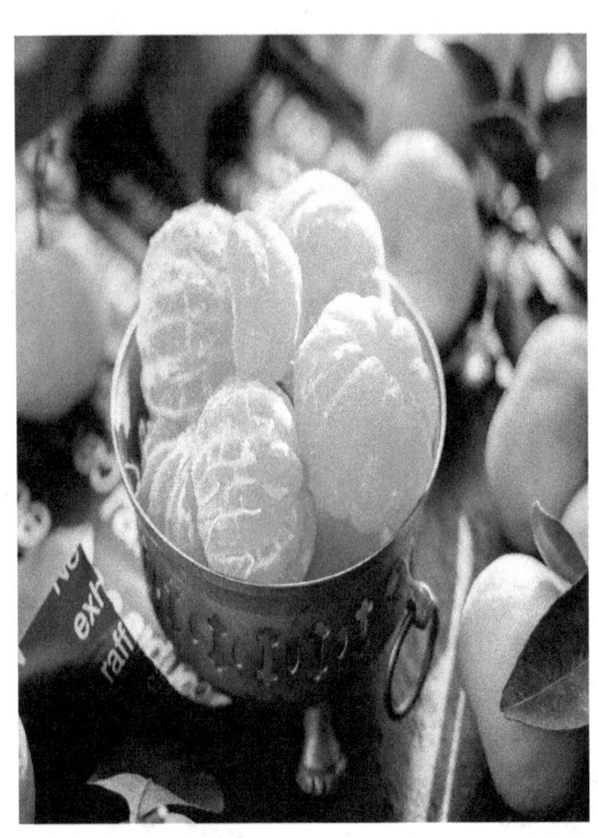
exh
raff

CHAPTER ONE

Why Juice?

Choosing juice can be a healthy and refreshing option, packed with vitamins and antioxidants. Its natural sweetness makes it a flavorful alternative to sugary beverages. Additionally, juice offers versatility—whether enjoyed on its own or used as a base for creative cocktails or mocktails. Opting for juice aligns with a balanced lifestyle, promoting hydration and supporting overall well-being

Benefits of juicing

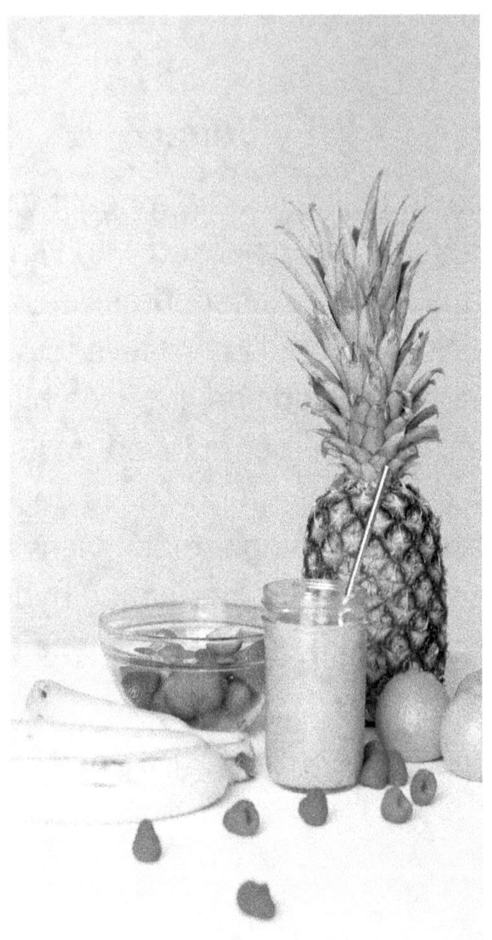

Juicing offers several potential benefits:

1. **Increased Nutrient Absorption**: Juicing extracts liquid from fruits and vegetables, providing a concentrated source of vitamins, minerals, and antioxidants, which can be absorbed more efficiently than whole foods.
2. **Enhanced Hydration**: Juices are rich in water content, contributing to hydration and supporting overall bodily functions.
3. **Digestive Health**: Juicing may aid digestion by breaking down plant fibers, making nutrients more accessible and reducing the strain on the digestive system.
4. **Weight Management:** [4] a radiant complexion.

5. **Detoxification**: While the body naturally detoxifies, some claim that certain juices can support the liver and kidneys in eliminating toxins, although scientific evidence is limited.
6. **Increased Energy Levels**: Nutrient-rich juices may provide a quick energy boost without the need for caffeine or sugary drinks.
7. **Alkalizing Properties**: Some proponents argue that juicing can help maintain a more alkaline environment in the body, potentially reducing the risk of certain health issues.
8. **Convenient Nutrient Intake**: Juicing offers a convenient way to consume a variety of fruits and vegetables, especially for those who find it challenging to eat enough whole produce.

It's essential to note that while juicing has its benefits, it's not a replacement for whole fruits and vegetables, as whole foods also provide important fiber. Additionally, individual responses to juicing can vary, and moderation is key.

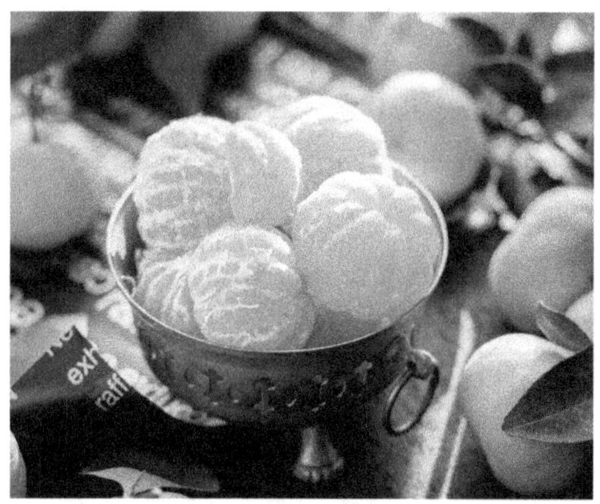

Getting Started

Creating healthy juices is a delightful journey that combines fresh, nutrient-rich ingredients with creativity.To get you started,consider these fundamentals:

1. **Choose Fresh Produce**:

Start with high-quality, fresh fruits and vegetables. Opt for a colorful variety to ensure a diverse range of nutrients. Wash and prep them thoroughly.

2. **Essential Tools**:

Invest in a good quality juicer. Centrifugal juicers are fast, while masticating juicers preserve more nutrients. You'll also need a sharp knife, cutting board, and a container for collecting the juice.

3. **Balanced Combinations**:

Create balanced flavors by combining fruits and vegetables. Consider sweet fruits like apples or oranges with leafy greens like kale or spinach. This not only enhances taste but also provides a broad spectrum of nutrients.

4. **Portion Control**:

Be mindful of portion sizes. While juices are nutrient-packed, excessive consumption may lead to a higher calorie intake. Aim for a balance that aligns with your dietary goals.

5. **Hydration Base**:

Water-rich fruits like cucumbers or watermelon make excellent hydrating bases. This not only adds volume but also contributes to overall hydration.

6. **Experiment with Herbs and Spices**:

Elevate your juice with herbs like mint or basil, and spices like ginger or turmeric. These additions not only enhance flavor but also bring additional health benefits.

7. **Juice Immediately:**

To retain maximum nutrients and freshness, consume the juice immediately after preparation. If storing is necessary, keep it in an airtight, dark container in the refrigerator for a short duration.

8. **Mindful Consumption:**

While juicing offers a concentrated source of nutrients, it's important to complement it with a well-rounded diet. Whole fruits and vegetables provide essential fiber that juices may lack.

9. **Clean Your Juicer:**

Clean your juicer promptly after use to prevent bacteria buildup. Regarding appreciate maintenance, consult the manufacturer's instructructions.

10. **Listen to Your Body:**

Keep an eye on how your body reacts to various combinations.

Everyone's taste preferences and nutritional needs vary, so customize your juices accordingly.

Embark on your juicing adventure with these basics, and soon you'll be creating delicious and nutritious concoctions tailored to your well-being

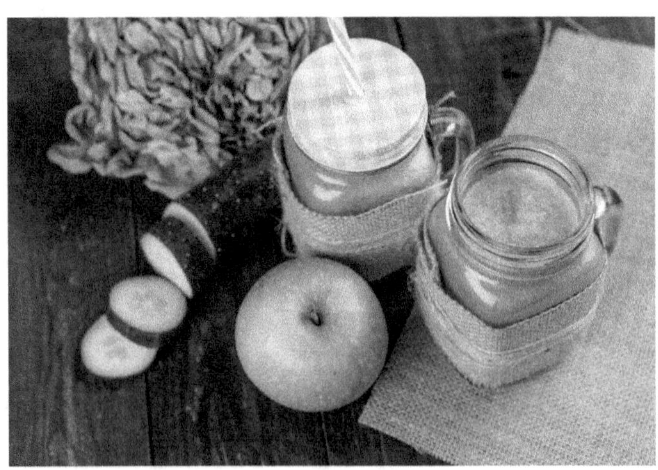

CHAPTER TWO

Choosing a juicer

When choosing a Juicer consider the following factors

1. **Type of Juicer**:
   - Centrifugal Juicers: Fast but may not extract as much juice from leafy greens.
   - Masticating Juicers (Cold Press): Slow, but efficient for leafy greens and retain more nutrients.
2. **Ease of Cleaning**:
   - Look for models with dishwasher-safe parts or easy-to-clean components.

3. **Juice Yield:**
    - Check reviews for feedback
      on how well the juicer
      extracts juice from different
      fruits and vegetables.
4. **Noise Level:**
    - Take into account the noise
      level,particularly if you intend
      to use it often.
5. **Juice Quality:**
    - Ensure the juicer produces
      high-quality juice with
      minimal oxidation for better
      taste and nutrition.
6. **Size of Feed Chute:**
    - A larger chute reduces prep
      time as it can accommodate
      whole or large pieces of
      fruits and vegetables.
7. **Motor Power:**
    - Higher wattage usually
      indicates a more powerful

motor, which can handle tougher produce.

8. **Build Quality**:
   - Choose a juicer with durable materials to ensure longevity.
9. **Versatility**:
   - Some juicers can also make nut butter, sorbet, or pasta. Consider if you want a multi-functional appliance.
10. **Pulp Ejection**:
    - Check if the juicer has an effective pulp ejection system for continuous juicing.
11. **Brand Reputation**:
    - Research and choose reputable brands known for quality juicers.

12. **Budget**:
    - Set a budget and find a juicer that meets your requirements within that range.
13. **Warranty**:
    - Ensure the juicer comes with a warranty for peace of mind.
14. **User Reviews**:
    - Read customer reviews to get insights into real-world experiences with the juicer model you're interested in.
15. **Size and Storage**:
    - Take the juicer's size into consideration, particularly if your counter space is at a premium

16. **Safety Features**:
    - Look for safety features like overload protection or a locking mechanism.
    -

By considering these factors, you can narrow down your options and find a juicer that suits your specific needs and preferences.

Essential Ingredients

For a basic and nutritious juice, consider a combination of fruits and vegetables. Here's a versatile list of ingredients:

Leafy Greens:

Spinach
Kale
Swiss chard

Fruits:

Apples
Oranges
Berries (strawberries, blueberries,
raspberries)

Citrus:

Lemons
Limes
Grapefruits

Root Vegetables:

Carrots
Beets
Cucumbers

Celery

Herbs:

Mint
Parsley
Ginger

Adjust proportions based on your taste preferences, and experiment with different combinations for variety and nutritional benefits.

Safety Tips and basic juicing Techniques

Safety Tips for Juicing:

Wash fruits and vegetables thoroughly
before juicing to remove pesticides and
contaminants.

Keep your knife and Cutting Board clean
to avoid cross-contamination
Check for any spoiled or moldy produce
and discard it.

Follow proper hygiene by washing your
hands
before handling ingredients and
equipment.
Keep juicing equipment, such as blades
and containers, clean and sanitized.

Unplug the juicer before assembling or
disassembling parts for cleaning.

Be cautious when handling sharp blades; use a tool or a brush for cleaning.

Store leftover juice in airtight containers in the refrigerator to prevent bacterial growth.

Be mindful of allergies and sensitivities when combining different ingredients.

Basic Juicing Techniques:

Choose Fresh Ingredients: Select ripe and fresh fruits and vegetables for the best flavor and nutritional value.

Preparation: Wash and chop ingredients into smaller pieces suitable for your juicer.

Layer Ingredients: Alternate soft and hard ingredients to optimize juicing .

Leafy Greens: Roll leafy greens into tight bundles before juicing to extract more juice.

Citrus Peel: If using citrus fruits, consider leaving some of the peel on for added flavor and nutrients.

Mix Flavors: Experiment with different combinations for unique and tasty juices.
Clean As You Go: Clean your juicer immediately after use to prevent residue buildup

.

Pulp Utilization: Repurpose leftover pulp in recipes like soups, smoothies, or baked goods.

Drink Fresh: Consume the juice immediately to maximize freshness and nutritional benefits.
Enjoy your juicing experience, and stay safe!

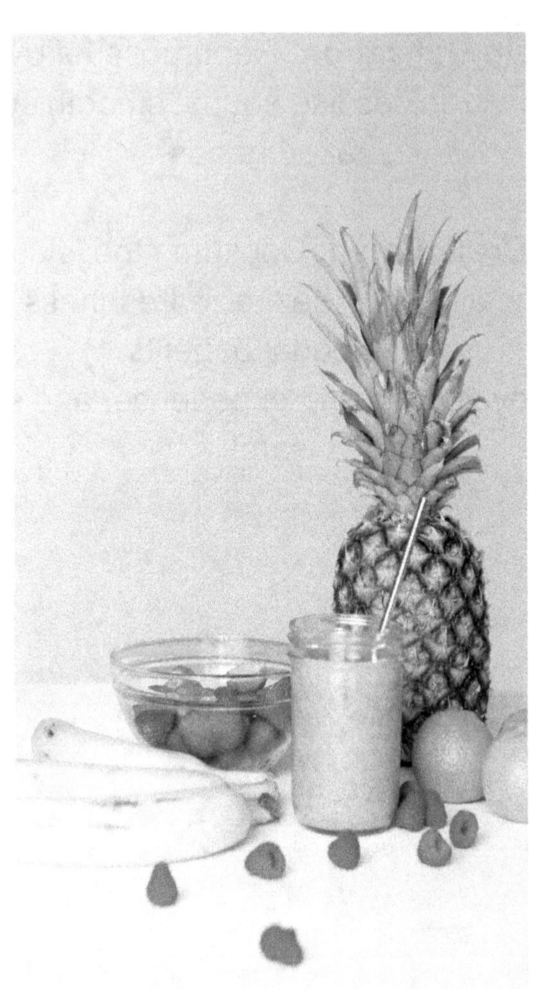

CHAPTER THREE

Washing and Preparing Produce

Washing and preparing produce for juicing is a crucial step to ensure the safety and quality of your juice. Follow these detailed guidelines to make the most of your juicing experience:

Selecting Fresh Produce:

Choose fresh, ripe fruits and vegetables for optimal flavor and nutritional content. Inspect produce for any signs of spoilage or damage before purchasing.

Organic Produce:

If you want to reduce your exposure to
pesticides, try buying organic fruits .
If using conventional produce, wash
them thoroughly to reduce pesticide
residues.

Basic Washing:

Rinse all fruits and vegetables under
cool, running water. Use a gentle stream
to avoid bruising delicate items.
Use a clean produce brush for items
with thicker skins, such as cucumbers or
carrots.

Leafy Greens:

Separate leaves of leafy greens, like
kale or spinach.
Immerse them in a bowl of water and
gently agitate to remove dirt.
Rinse under running water, ensuring
thorough cleaning.

Root Vegetables:

Scrub root vegetables like carrots or
beets with a brush to remove soil.
Trim off the ends and any blemishes.

Citrus Fruits:

Wash citrus fruits thoroughly, as their
peels might be used in juicing.
Consider using a natural produce wash
or a mixture of water and vinegar for
added cleanliness.

Berries:

Soak berries in a bowl of water to
dislodge dirt.
Use a salad spinner or a paper towel to
gently pat them dry.

Peeling and Pitting:

Remove peels from fruits like oranges or
pineapples if you prefer a smoother
texture.
Pit fruits like cherries or peaches before
juicing.

Seeds and Cores:

Remove seeds from fruits such as
apples or watermelon.
Cut out cores or tough parts that may
affect the juicing process.

Storing Prepared Produce:

Once cleaned and prepared, store the produce in a clean, airtight container in the refrigerator until ready to juice. Avoid cutting fruits too far in advance to prevent nutrient loss.

Maintaining Hygiene:

Wash hands thoroughly before handling produce.
Clean and sanitize cutting boards, knives, and juicer parts to prevent cross-contamination.
By following these steps, you ensure that your produce is clean, safe, and ready to be transformed into a refreshing and nutritious juice.

Juicing Methods

Juicing is a popular way to consume fruits and vegetables in a concentrated form. Here's a basic guide to get you started:

Equipment:

Juicer: Choose between a centrifugal or masticating juicer based on your preferences.
Knife and Cutting Board: For preparing fruits and vegetables.

Glass or Container: To collect the juice.

Steps:

Choose Fresh Produce:

Use a variety of fruits and vegetables for a well-rounded juice.
Wash them thoroughly to remove pesticides and dirt.

Preparation:

Peel and cut large fruits into smaller pieces.
Remove seeds or pits from fruits if necessary.
Trim and cut vegetables as needed.

Juicing:

Follow your juicer's instructions for assembly.
Feed the produce through the juicer one piece at a time.

For leafy greens, roll them into compact bundles to extract more juice.

Mixing Flavors:

Experiment with different combinations
for unique flavors.
Consider adding herbs like mint or
ginger for extra zest.

Serve Immediately:

Freshly squeezed juice is most nutritious
when consumed right away.
If you need to store it, use airtight
containers and refrigerate for up to 24
hours.

Clean Your Juicer:

Disassemble the juicer and clean each
part thoroughly after use.
This prevents residue buildup and
ensures longevity.

Tips:

Balance sweet and tangy fruits to avoid
overly sweet or sour juices.
Use a range of hues to represent
different types of nutrients.
Drink juice in moderation as part of a
balanced diet.
Remember, while juicing can be a
convenient way to increase your intake
of fruits and vegetables, it's essential to
also consume whole, fiber-rich produce
for overall health.

Mixing Flavors and popular juice Recipes

Mixing flavors in juice recipes can lead to unique and delightful combinations. Here are some popular juice recipes that showcase the art of flavor blending:

Tropical Bliss:

Ingredients: Pineapple, mango, coconut water, and a hint of lime.
Method: Blend fresh pineapple chunks and mango slices with coconut water. Add a splash of lime juice for a refreshing tropical twist.

Berry Citrus Fusion:

Ingredients: Mixed berries (strawberries, blueberries, raspberries), orange, and a touch of mint.

Method: Combine the vibrant flavors of mixed berries with freshly squeezed orange juice. Garnish with a few mint leaves for a burst of freshness.

Cucumber Melon Refresher:

Ingredients: Cucumber, watermelon, mint, and a squeeze of lemon. Method: Blend cucumber and watermelon chunks, then add a handful of mint leaves and a splash of lemon juice. This recipe is hydrating and invigorating.

Green Goddess Elixir:

Ingredients: Kale, apple, cucumber, celery, and ginger.

Method: Juice kale, apple, cucumber, celery, and a small piece of ginger to create a nutrient-packed green juice. This combination offers a balance of sweetness and earthiness.

Citrus Mint Medley:

Ingredients: Oranges, grapefruit, lime, and fresh mint.
Method: Extract juice from oranges, grapefruit, and lime. Mix the citrus juices and add finely chopped mint leaves. This recipe is zesty with a cooling minty finish.

Carrot Ginger Zing:

Ingredients: Carrots, apples, ginger, and a hint of turmeric.

Method: Juice carrots and apples together, then add freshly grated ginger and a pinch of turmeric for a vibrant and immune-boosting concoction.Remember, experimenting with proportions allows you to tailor these recipes to your taste preferences. Start with small quantities, taste as you go, and enjoy the journey of discovering your favorite personalized juice blends.

CHAPTER FOUR

Energizing Green Juice

Energizing Green Juice is a nutrient-packed beverage made from a blend of fresh green vegetables and

fruits. Typically, ingredients like kale, spinach, cucumber, celery, and green apples are combined to create a refreshing and health-boosting drink. This juice is renowned for its high content of vitamins, minerals, and antioxidants, promoting energy levels, aiding in digestion, and supporting overall well-being. It's a popular choice among those seeking a natural way to rejuvenate and revitalize their body.

Energizing Green Juice Recipe:

Ingredients:

2 cups of kale leaves
1 cucumber
1 green apple
1 lemon (peeled)
1-inch piece of ginger
1 celery stalk
1 cup of spinach leaves
1/2 cup of parsley
1/2 cup of mint leaves
One or two cups of water (diluted to desired consistency)

Instructions:

Prepare Ingredients:
Wash all the vegetables and fruits thoroughly. Cut the cucumber, apple, and celery into smaller pieces to fit into the juicer.

Juicing:

Start by juicing the kale, spinach, cucumber, green apple, lemon, ginger, celery, parsley, and mint leaves. Make sure to alternate between leafy greens and harder vegetables to optimize the juicing process.

Adjust Consistency:
Depending on your preference, you can add water gradually while juicing to achieve the desired consistency. Some prefer a thicker juice, while others may like it more diluted.

Mix Well:
Once the juicing is complete, give the mixture a good stir to ensure an even distribution of flavors.

Serve Immediately:
Freshly made juice is at its peak in terms of both taste and nutritional value. Serve the green juice immediately to enjoy the maximum benefits.

Additional Tips:

To suit your taste preferences, experiment with the ingredient quantities.
Adjust sweetness and tartness by adding more or less apple and lemon.

For an extra boost, you can add a scoop of chia seeds or a splash of coconut water.
Consider using organic produce for a cleaner and more nutrient-dense juice.

This Energizing Green Juice is packed with vitamins, minerals, and antioxidants, providing a refreshing and nutritious way to start your day or boost your energy levels.

Citrus Bliss

Citrus Bliss is a delightful blend of citrus fruits, typically including oranges, lemons, and limes. When juicing, ensure your fruits are fresh and ripe for the best flavor. Experiment with different ratios to find your preferred citrus combination. Consider adding a touch of sweetness with a splash of pineapple or a hint of mint for an extra refreshing twist. Adjusting the balance between sweet and tart can tailor the juice to your taste preferences. Enjoy the vibrant burst of flavor that Citrus Bliss brings to your homemade juice!

To make a refreshing Citrus Bliss juice, gather the following ingredients:

Ingredients:

Oranges
Grapefruits
Lemons
Limes
Sugar or sweetener (optional)
Ice cubes (optional)

Instructions:

Wash and peel the citrus fruits. Remove any seeds or pith.
Cut the fruits into manageable pieces, making it easier to juice.
Use a citrus juicer or a manual juicing method to extract the juice from each fruit.
Combine the freshly squeezed juice in a pitch

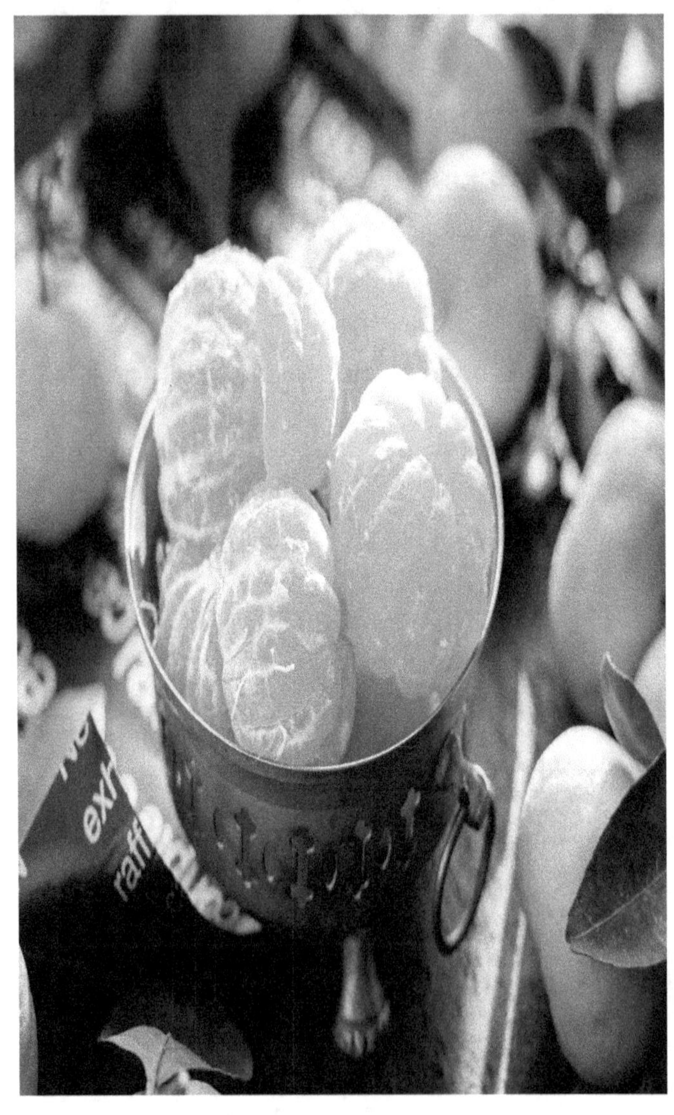

er, adjusting the ratios to your taste
preference.
If desired, add sugar or a sweetener of
your choice to enhance the sweetness.

Stir well until the sweetener is dissolved.
To enjoy a cool,refreshing
drink,refrigerate the juice.
Optionally, add ice cubes to individual
servings for an extra cool experience.

Serve the Citrus Bliss juice in your
favorite glass and enjoy the burst of
citrus flavors.
Feel free to experiment with different
citrus fruit combinations and sweetness
levels to tailor the juice to your liking.

Beginners Berry Blend

Customizing Your Juices

Berry Blend juices are a delightful way to combine the goodness of various berries into a refreshing drink. To customize your juice, start with a base of berries like strawberries, blueberries, and raspberries. Experiment with ratios to find your preferred taste.

Consider adding a splash of citrus for a zesty twist or a hint of sweetness with apple or pear. Don't forget to balance flavors - a touch of mint can add freshness. Play with textures by blending in ice or yogurt. Start simple, then refine your recipe based on personal preference. Enjoy your personalized berry blend!

Beginners Berry Blend

Berry Blast:

Ingredients: 1 cup strawberries, 1/2 cup blueberries, 1/2 cup raspberries, 1 cup blackberries.

Instructions: Blend all the berries together with water or your preferred liquid base. If desired,add some honey or a sweetener.

Tropical Berry Paradise:

Ingredients: 1 cup mixed berries, 1/2 cup pineapple chunks, 1/2 cup mango chunks.

Instructions: Blend the mixed berries, pineapple, and mango for a refreshing tropical twist. Consider adding coconut water for extra flavor.

Citrus Berry Splash:

Ingredients: 1 cup mixed berries, 1 orange (peeled), 1/2 cup strawberries, 1 tablespoon lime juice.
Instructions: Combine berries, peeled orange, and lime juice in a blender. Blend until smooth. Adjust sweetness with honey if needed.

Customization Tips:

Base Liquid: Choose a liquid base like water, coconut water, almond milk, or even green tea.

Sweeteners: Adjust sweetness with honey, agave syrup, or a natural sweetener.

Texture Boost: Add texture with chia seeds, flaxseeds, or oats.
Green Boost: Incorporate spinach or kale for added nutrients without altering the flavor much.

Protein Kick: Blend in Greek yogurt, protein powder, or nut butter for a protein boost.

Spices: Enhance flavor with a pinch of cinnamon, ginger, or mint leaves.
Ice: For a chilled and slushy texture, add ice cubes to your liking.

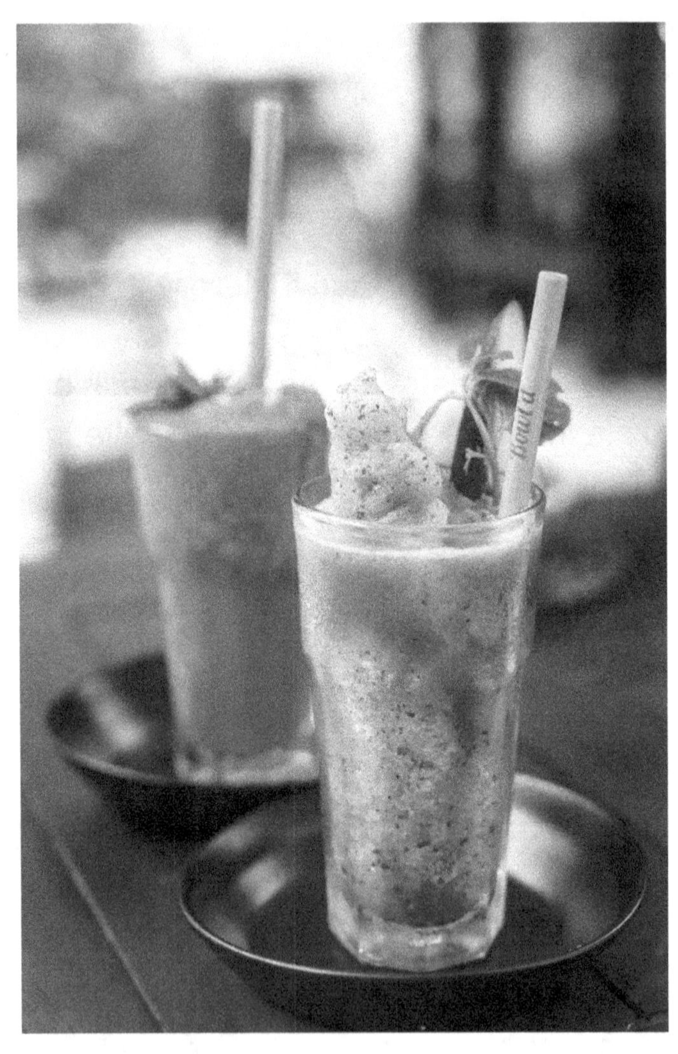

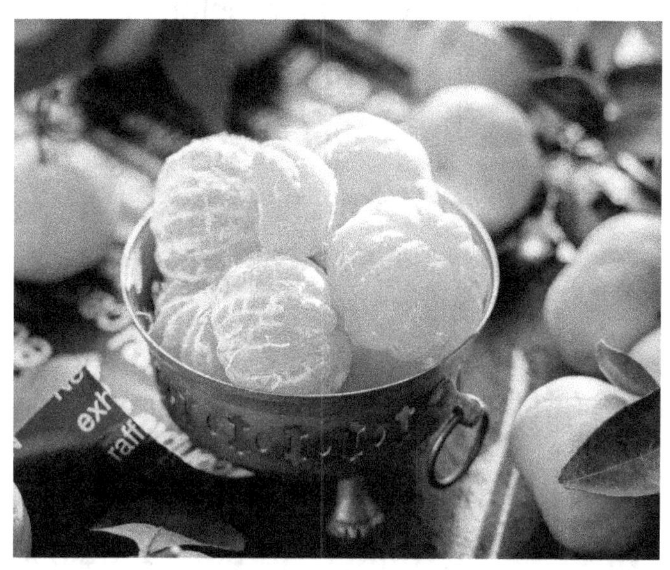

CHAPTER FIVE

Tailoring to Dietary Needs

Understand Dietary Needs: Begin by understanding the dietary needs of the individual. Consider factors like allergies, intolerances, and any specific dietary restrictions.

Consult with a Professional: If the person has specific health concerns or dietary requirements, it's advisable to consult with a healthcare professional or a nutritionist to ensure the juicing plan meets their needs.

Choose the Right Ingredients: Select fruits and vegetables that align with the individual's dietary requirements. For example, if someone is on a low-sugar diet, opt for vegetables with lower sugar content.

Address Allergies and Intolerances: Avoid ingredients that may trigger allergies or intolerances. Nuts,dairy products, and several fruits are common sources of allergies. Substitute with safe alternatives.

Balance Macronutrients: Ensure a balanced mix of macronutrients - proteins, carbohydrates, and fats. Incorporate ingredients like leafy greens, seeds, and nuts to provide a well-rounded nutritional profile.

Monitor Sugar Intake: For individuals with diabetes or those watching their sugar intake, focus on low-glycemic fruits and vegetables. Limit the use of high-sugar fruits like pineapples or mangos.

Include Fiber: Fiber is essential for digestion and can help stabilize blood sugar levels. Keep the pulp in the juice or add it back in to increase fiber content.

Hydration: Consider using coconut water or herbal teas as a base instead of high-sugar fruit juices to maintain hydration without excess sugar.

Experiment with Nutrient-Rich Additions: Add nutrient-dense ingredients like spirulina, chia seeds, or flaxseeds to enhance the nutritional value of the juice.

Portion Control: Be mindful of portion sizes, especially if the individual is on a specific calorie-controlled diet. Juices can be calorie-dense, so moderation is key.

Monitor Electrolytes: If someone has specific electrolyte needs, incorporate ingredients like celery or coconut water to help maintain electrolyte balance.

Keep it Varied: Introduce a variety of fruits and vegetables to ensure a diverse nutrient intake. This helps prevent nutrient deficiencies and keeps the diet interesting.

Consider Digestive Health: Include ingredients that support digestive health, such as ginger or probiotics, especially if the individual has specific digestive concerns.

Remember, individual needs vary, and it's crucial to tailor the juicing plan based on the specific dietary requirements and health goals of the person in question.

Adjusting Sweetness and Thickness Health

Considerations

Adjusting Sweetness and Thickness in Juicing:

Adjusting Sweetness:

Choose Sweet Fruits: Incorporate naturally sweet fruits like apples, pineapples, or berries into your juice for sweetness.

Balance with Greens: Counteract the sweetness with leafy greens like kale or spinach to add nutritional value and reduce overall sugar content.

Citrus Zest: Enhance sweetness without added sugar by incorporating citrus zest, such as lemon or orange, for a burst of flavor.

Adjusting Thickness:

Use Thickening Agents: Add ingredients like avocados, chia seeds, or bananas to increase the thickness and creaminess of your juice.
Include Fibrous Fruits: Opt for fibrous fruits like mangoes or papayas, as they contribute to a thicker texture.

Experiment with Vegetables: Vegetables like carrots and beets can add substance to your juice without compromising nutritional value.

Health Considerations:

Monitor Sugar Intake:
Choose Whole Fruits: Favor whole fruits over fruit juices to retain fiber, which helps regulate blood sugar levels.

Limit Added Sweeteners: Minimize or avoid adding additional sweeteners to maintain the natural sweetness of fruits.

Consider Low-Glycemic Options: Opt for low-glycemic fruits like berries to reduce the impact on blood sugar.

Maximize Nutrient Intake:
Include a Variety of Colors: Incorporate a diverse range of fruits and vegetables with different colors to ensure a broad spectrum of nutrients.

Prioritize Leafy Greens: Make leafy greens a significant part of your juice for essential vitamins and minerals. Rotate Ingredients: Rotate your ingredients regularly to expose your body to various nutrients and prevent monotony.

Personalize for Dietary Needs:

Consult with a Nutritionist: If you have specific health concerns or dietary restrictions, consult with a nutritionist to tailor your juice recipes accordingly.

Consider Allergies: Be mindful of any allergies or intolerances you may have and select ingredients that align with your health needs.
Monitor Portion Sizes: Even with healthy juices, moderation is key. Keep

an eye on portion amounts to keep your diet balanced.
Remember to enjoy your juices in moderation and consider individual health conditions when adjusting sweetness and thickness.

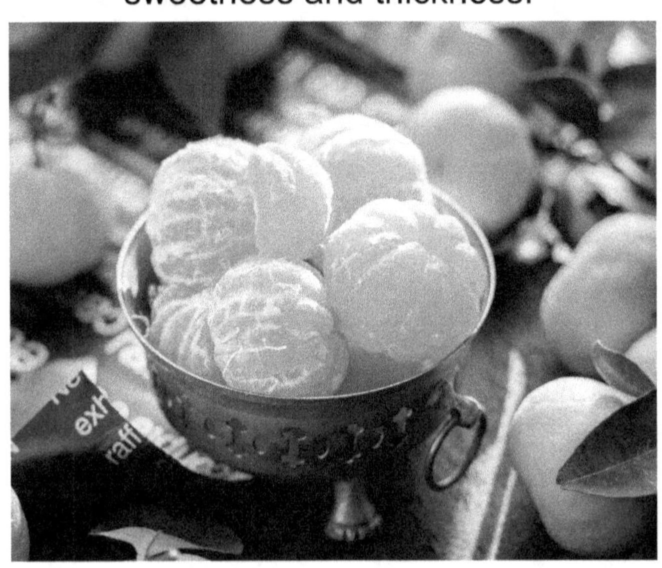

CHAPTER SIX

Nutritional Benefits

Juicing can offer various nutritional benefits, providing a convenient way to increase your intake of essential vitamins, minerals, and antioxidants.

The nutritional advantages are outlined as follows:

Abundance of Vitamins and Minerals:

Fruits and vegetables used in juicing are rich in vitamins such as A, C, and K, as well as essential minerals like potassium and magnesium.

Antioxidant Boost:

Juices from colorful fruits and vegetables contain antioxidants like flavonoids and carotenoids, which help combat oxidative stress and reduce inflammation in the body.

Hydration:

Juicing contributes to hydration as fruits and vegetables have high water content.

Water consumption is crucial for a number of bodily functions.

Digestive Health:

Fiber in fruits and vegetables supports digestive health. While juicing removes some fiber, leaving the pulp can provide additional fiber, promoting a healthy gut and regular bowel movements.

Immune System Support:

Vitamin C, present in citrus fruits like oranges and lemons, can enhance the immune system's function, helping the body fend off infections and illnesses.

Detoxification:

Some vegetables, like celery and beetroot, are believed to have detoxifying properties, supporting liver function and aiding the body's natural detox processes.

Increased Nutrient Absorption:

Juicing breaks down the cell walls of fruits and vegetables, making the nutrients more accessible for absorption, potentially increasing the bioavailability of certain vitamins and minerals.

Weight Management:

Juicing can be a part of a balanced diet for weight management, providing nutrient-dense options with lower calorie density. However, it's essential to maintain a diverse and balanced diet.

Improved Skin Health:

Nutrients like vitamin E and beta-carotene in fruits and vegetables contribute to healthier skin, promoting a radiant complexion and possibly slowing down the aging process.

Energy Boost:

The natural sugars in fruits can provide a quick energy boost, making juices a refreshing and revitalizing option, particularly when consumed in moderation.
While juicing offers numerous nutritional benefits, it's important to balance it with whole, unprocessed foods to ensure you get a variety of nutrients, including fiber. Additionally, be mindful of portion sizes and avoid excessive consumption of

juices high in natural sugars to maintain
a well-rounded and healthy diet.

Potential Pitfalls

Juicing can offer a convenient way to
increase your fruit and vegetable intake,
but it also comes with potential pitfalls.
Here are some considerations:

Loss of Fiber: Juicing extracts the liquid
from fruits and vegetables, leaving
behind the fiber. Fiber is crucial for
digestive health and can help regulate
blood sugar levels. Consuming only
juice may lead to a lack of essential
dietary fiber.

Caloric Intake: While juices are often considered healthy, they can be calorically dense, especially if they contain a high amount of fruits. This may contribute to excess calorie consumption, potentially leading to weight gain.

Sugar Content: Fruits contain natural sugars, and when juiced, the concentration of sugar in a serving can be much higher than eating whole fruits. Excessive sugar intake can contribute to various health issues, including insulin resistance and weight gain.

Nutrient Imbalance: Juicing may not provide a balanced mix of nutrients compared to consuming whole fruits and vegetables. For instance, the juicing process can lead to a loss of certain heat-sensitive vitamins and antioxidants.

Oxidation: Exposure to air during the juicing process can lead to oxidation, which may reduce the nutritional value of the juice. Drinking freshly made juice immediately is ideal to minimize this effect.

Hydration Misconception: While juice contains water, it should not replace plain water as the primary source of hydration. Drinking too much juice without sufficient water intake can contribute to dehydration.

Expense: Regularly juicing can be costly, as it requires a significant amount of fruits and vegetables to produce a small quantity of juice. Some people may find this expense to be prohibitive.

Digestive Issues: Consuming large quantities of certain fruits and vegetables in juice form may lead to digestive discomfort for some people. It may result in symptoms like diarrhea, gas,or bloating.

Potential for Contamination: Freshly squeezed juices can be a breeding ground for bacteria if not handled and stored properly. It's important to clean juicing equipment thoroughly and store juice in a hygienic manner.

Sustainability Concerns: The demand for large quantities of produce for juicing can have environmental implications, contributing to issues like deforestation, pesticide use, and excessive water consumption.

To mitigate these pitfalls, it's advisable to complement juicing with a well-rounded diet that includes a variety of whole fruits, vegetables, and other nutrient-rich foods. Moderation and balance are key for a healthy approach to juicing.

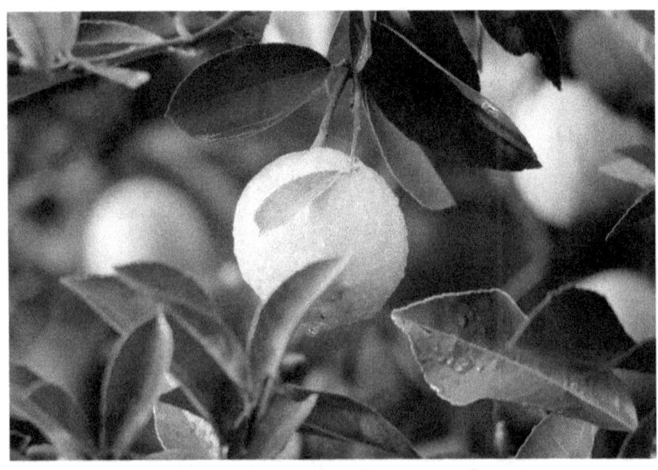

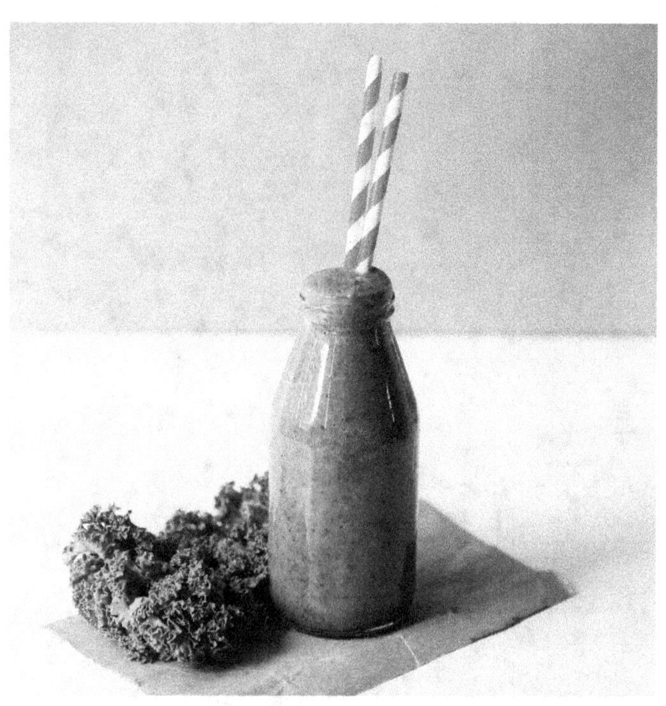

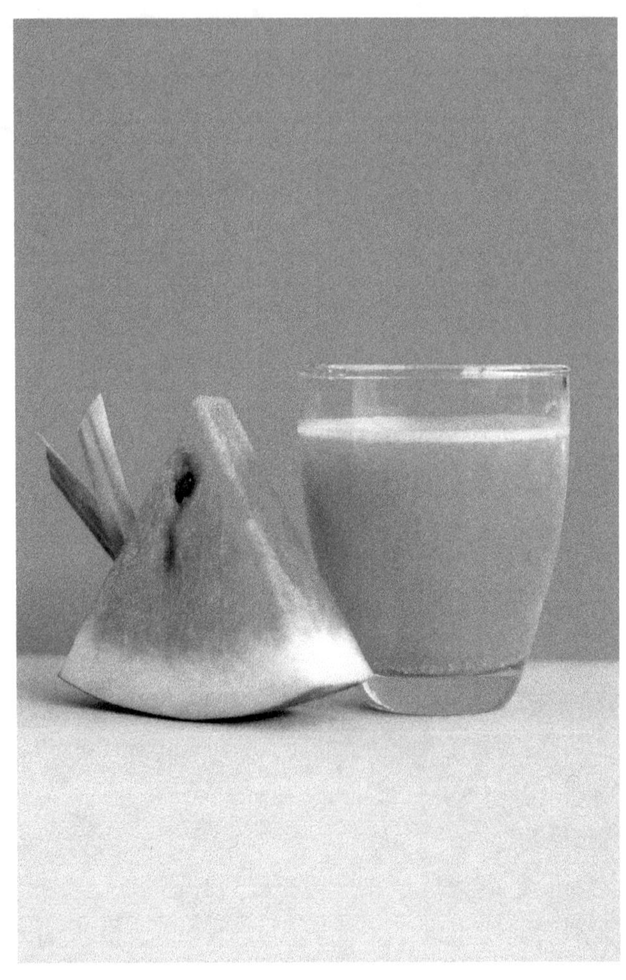

CHAPTER SEVEN

Meal Replacement or Supplement?

Meal replacement or supplements can be a convenient addition to a juicing regimen, providing essential nutrients when used wisely.

Meal Replacement:

Nutrient Balance: Opt for a meal replacement that offers a balanced mix of macronutrients (proteins, carbohydrates, and fats) and micronutrients (vitamins and minerals). This ensures you're getting a well-rounded nutritional intake.

Caloric Content: Consider the caloric content of the meal replacement in relation to your overall daily calorie needs. It's essential to maintain a healthy calorie balance to meet your goals, whether it's weight loss, maintenance, or muscle gain.

Quality Ingredients: Choose products with high-quality ingredients, avoiding excessive sugars, artificial additives, and preservatives. Look for natural sources of protein, like whey or plant-based options, and whole-food-based carbohydrates.

Personal Goals: Tailor your choice based on your specific health and fitness goals. Some meal replacements are designed for weight loss, while others focus on muscle gain or overall nutrition.

Nutrient Gaps: Supplements can help fill nutritional gaps that may arise from a juicing-centric diet. Consider adding vitamins, minerals, or specific nutrients that may be lacking in your juice blends.

Protein Supplements: If your juicing plan lacks sufficient protein, consider incorporating protein supplements. This is particularly important if you're aiming for muscle maintenance or growth.

Omega-3 Fatty Acids: While juicing can provide a variety of nutrients, it might be deficient in omega-3 fatty acids. Omega-3 supplements, such as fish oil or algae-based supplements, can support overall health, especially brain and heart health.

Consultation: Before adding any supplements or meal replacements, consult with a healthcare professional or a nutritionist. They can provide personalized advice based on your individual health needs and dietary requirements.

Remember that while meal replacements and supplements can be beneficial, whole foods should remain the foundation of your diet. They provide a wide array of nutrients and fiber that may be lacking in processed options. Always prioritize a balanced and varied diet for optimal health.

Juicing for Detox: A Comprehensive Guide

Juicing has gained popularity as a method for detoxifying the body, providing a boost of nutrients, and promoting overall well-being.

Here's a detailed guide on juicing for detox, including recipes and troubleshooting tips.

1. **Understanding Detoxification**: Detoxification is the process of eliminating toxins from the body, and juicing is believed to support this by

providing essential nutrients while allowing the digestive system to rest.

2. **Choosing the Right Ingredients**:

Opt for organic fruits and vegetables to minimize exposure to pesticides. Include a variety of colors to ensure a broad spectrum of nutrients. Common detoxifying ingredients include kale, spinach, celery, cucumber, lemon, ginger, and beets.

3. **Basic Detox Juice Recipe:**

1 cucumber
2 stalks of celery
1 cup of spinach
1/2 lemon (peeled)
1 inch of ginger
1 apple (cored)

4. Troubleshooting Tips:

Bitter Taste: Add a sweeter fruit like apple or pear to balance the flavors.

Thick Texture: Strain the juice or dilute with water for a smoother consistency.

Foam: Remove foam by skimming the top with a spoon or using a fine mesh strainer.

5. Detox Juice Variations:

Green Goddess Juice:

Kale
Green apple
Cucumber
Lemon

Mint leaves
Beet Blast Juice:

Beets
Carrots
Apple
Lemon
Ginger

Citrus Sunshine Juice:

Oranges
Grapefruit
Pineapple
Mint

6. Incorporating Detox into Your Routine:

Start with one juice a day and gradually increase.

Stay hydrated with water throughout the day.
Combine juicing with a balanced diet for optimal results.

7. **Precautions and Considerations**:

Before starting any detox treatment, see a medical professional.
Monitor sugar intake, as some fruits are high in natural sugars.
Detox is not a long-term solution; consider it as part of a healthy lifestyle.
Juicing for detox can be a refreshing addition to your wellness routine.
Experiment with different recipes, listen to your body, and enjoy the benefits of nourishing your system with vibrant, nutrient-rich juices.

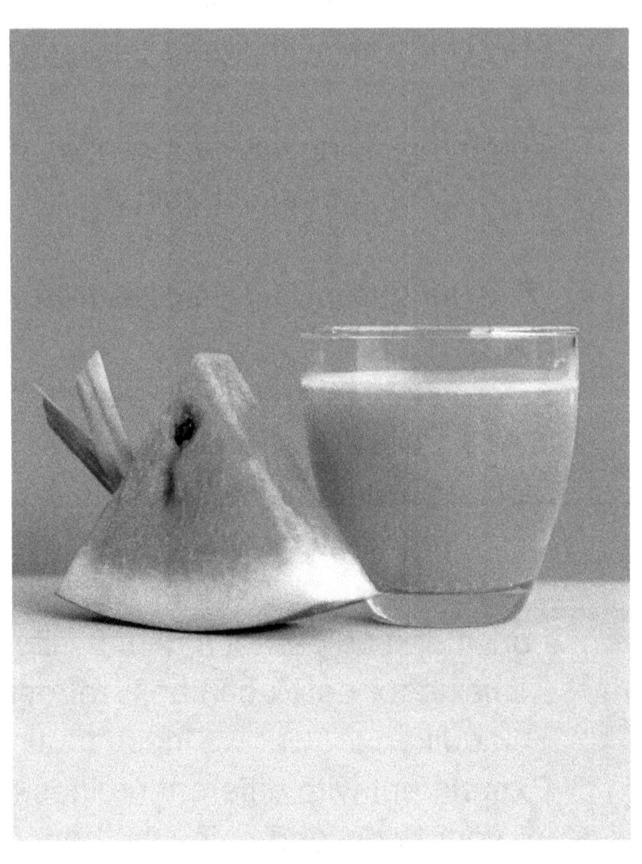

CHAPTER EIGHT

Common Juicing Issues

common juicing issues and their remedies:

Clogging:

Issue: Produce pulp may clog the juicer, reducing efficiency.

Remedy: Cut fibrous fruits and vegetables into smaller pieces. Alternate between soft and hard items to help prevent clogging.

Foaming:

Issue: Excessive foam in the juice can affect taste and quality.

Remedy: Slowly feed ingredients into the juicer. Skim foam off the top or let it settle before consuming.

Bitter Taste:

Issue: Some juices may turn out bitter, especially with certain greens.

Remedy: Balance bitter greens with sweeter fruits like apples or citrus. Adjust quantities for a more palatable taste.

Overheating:

Issue: Continuous juicing may cause the machine to overheat.

Remedy: Allow the juicer to cool down between batches. Follow recommended usage times in the user manual.

Jamming:

Issue: Pieces of produce may get stuck, leading to jamming.
Remedy: Use a plunger or reverse function (if available) to unclog. Avoid forcing ingredients into the juicer.

Leakage:

Issue: Juicer may leak juice or pulp during operation.
Remedy: Check for loose parts or misalignment. Ensure all components are securely locked in place before use.

Inconsistent Juice Extraction:

Issue: Uneven extraction of juice from different ingredients.

Remedy: Rotate or mix ingredients to improve consistency. Adjust the juicer settings based on the hardness of produce.

Cleaning Challenges:

Issue: Cleaning the juicer can be time-consuming and challenging.

Remedy: Clean the juicer immediately after use to prevent residue buildup. For cleaning and disassembly, adhere to the manufacturer's recommendations.

Limited Juice Yield:

Issue: Not extracting the maximum juice from fruits and vegetables.

Remedy: Experiment with different combinations. Some produce may require additional pressure or a slower juicing speed.

Noise:

Issue: Juicer produces excessive noise during operation.

Remedy: Check for loose parts or misalignment. To reduce vibrations, set the juicer on a sturdy surface. Remember to consult your juicer's manual for specific troubleshooting tips and maintenance guidelines.

Maintenance and Cleaning FAQs

How often should I clean my juicer?

Regular cleaning is crucial to maintain optimal performance. Clean your juicer after each use to prevent residue buildup.

Can I put my juicer parts in the dishwasher?

Check the manufacturer's instructions. While some parts may be dishwasher-safe, it's often recommended to hand wash them to preserve the longevity of certain components.

What's the best way to clean the mesh filter?

Use a soft brush or sponge to scrub away pulp residue. Soaking the filter in warm, soapy water can help loosen stubborn particles.

Is it necessary to disassemble the juicer for cleaning?

Yes, thorough cleaning involves disassembling the juicer. Remove all removable parts and clean each one separately to ensure no leftover pulp or juice.

How do I clean the juicer's feed chute?

Wipe down the feed chute with a damp cloth after each use to prevent dried-on residue. If needed, use a small brush to clean hard-to-reach areas.

Can I use cleaning agents on my juicer?

Stick to mild, natural cleaning agents like a mixture of water and vinegar. Avoid harsh chemicals that may affect the taste of your juice.

What if I notice stains on the juicer components?
Stains from fruits and vegetables are common. To remove them, soak the affected parts in a solution of water and baking soda or lemon juice.

How often should I replace juicer parts?
Refer to your juicer's manual for specific guidelines. Generally, replace parts like blades or filters if you notice signs of wear or reduced efficiency.

Can I store my juicer with leftover pulp inside?
It's not recommended. Remove and discard leftover pulp after juicing, as leaving it in the juicer can lead to mold growth and unpleasant odors.

Any tips for quick and efficient cleaning?
Clean immediately after use to prevent drying of pulp. Keep a dedicated brush for juicer cleaning to make the process more efficient.

Remember, proper maintenance and cleaning not only ensure the longevity of your juicer but also contribute to the quality and taste of your freshly squeezed juices.

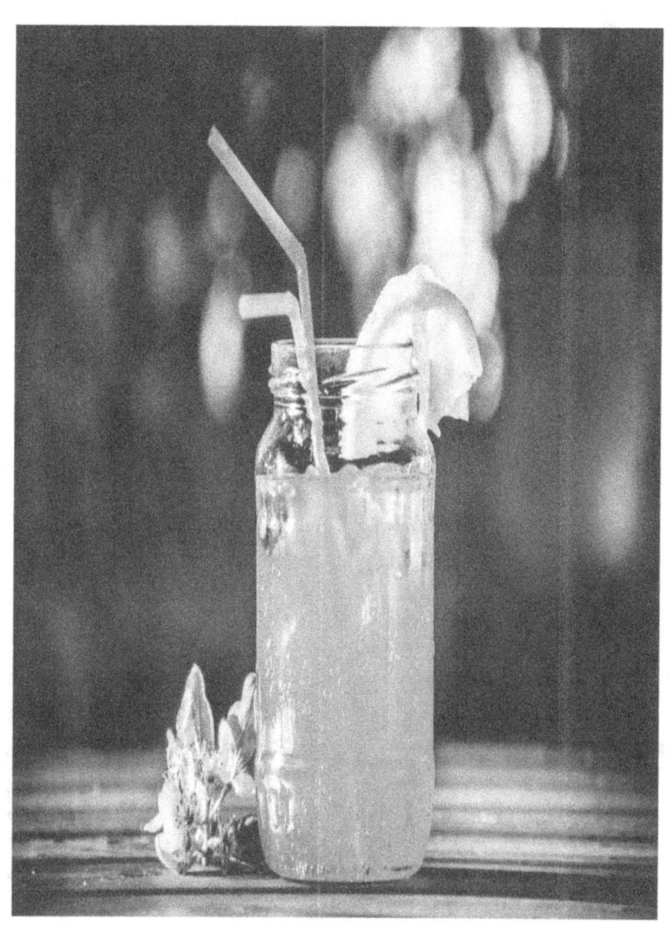

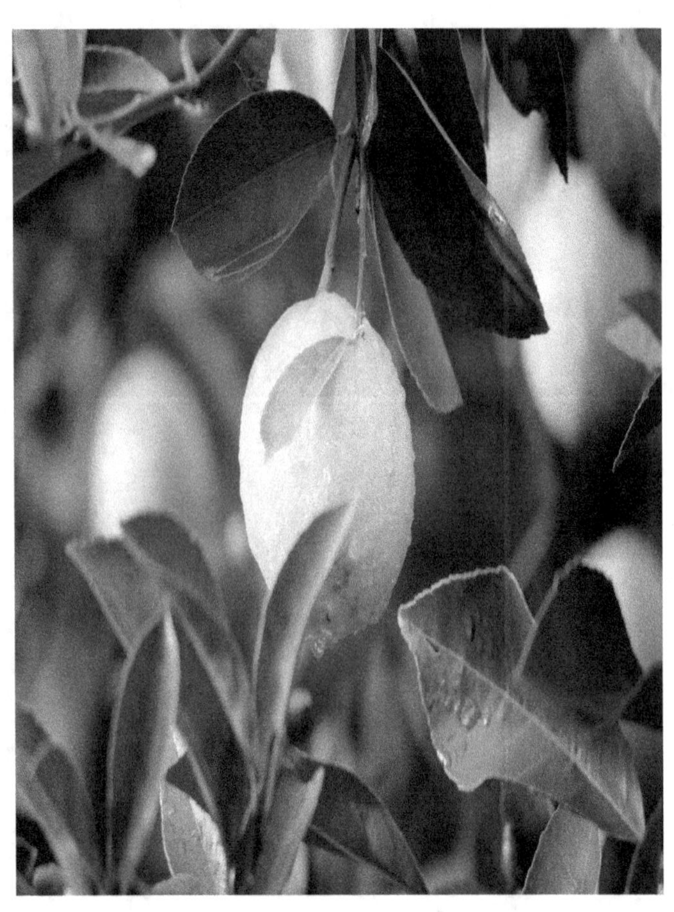

CHAPTER NINE

Addressing Common Questions

Here's a brief guide addressing common questions:

Why Juice?

Nutrient Absorption: Juicing allows for quick nutrient absorption as it removes fiber, making nutrients readily available.

Convenience: Provides an easy way to consume a variety of fruits and vegetables in a single glass.

Which Fruits and Vegetables are Best?

Diversity: Aim for a mix of colorful produce to ensure a broad spectrum of vitamins and minerals.

Balance: Include both fruits and vegetables, but be cautious of high sugar content in fruits.

What About Fiber?

Fiber Removal: Juicing extracts fiber, which can aid digestion, but it's essential to balance with whole foods to maintain fiber intake.

Is Juicing a Detox Method?

Limited Evidence: While some claim juicing detoxifies the body, scientific evidence is limited. A well-balanced diet supports natural detoxification processes.

How to Avoid Sugar Overload?

Limit High-Sugar Fruits: Be mindful of using too many high-sugar fruits. Include more vegetables to reduce overall sugar content.

Is Juicing a Meal Replacement?

Supplement, Not Replace: Juices can be a nutritious addition to your diet but should not replace whole meals. They lack essential proteins and fats.

Can I Juice Ahead of Time?

Freshness Matters: Freshly squeezed juice retains more nutrients. If storing, use airtight containers and consume within 24 hours to minimize nutrient loss.

What Equipment is Needed?

Juicer Selection: Choose a juicer based on your preferences – centrifugal for speed

or masticating for nutrient retention.
Consider ease of cleaning.

Are There Risks?

Caloric Intake: Juicing may reduce caloric intake, which can be a concern if not supplemented with enough calories from other sources.

Should I Cleanse with Juicing?

Consultation Advised: Consult a healthcare professional before embarking on a juice cleanse, as prolonged liquid diets may lack essential nutrients.
Remember, while juicing offers benefits, a balanced diet incorporating whole fruits and vegetables, along with diverse

nutrients, is crucial for overall health. For individualized guidance, always seek the opinion of a healthcare provider or nutritionist.

Celebrating Your Juicing Journey

Embarking on a juicing journey is not just about sipping nutritious concoctions; it's a celebration of vitality and well-being. Start by reflecting on your progress, noting how this venture has positively impacted your health. Whether it's increased energy, clearer skin, or better digestion, acknowledge and celebrate these achievements.

Create a ritual around your juicing experience. Dedicate a specific time each day to savor your freshly pressed juices, perhaps during sunrise or sunset. Consider incorporating mindful practices like deep breathing or gratitude reflection to enhance the holistic benefits of your routine.

Document your juicing journey through a journal or social media. Share your favorite recipes, the challenges you've overcome, and the moments of triumph. This not only reinforces your commitment but also inspires others on similar paths.

Host a juicing party or invite friends to join your celebration. Share the joy of discovering new flavors and experimenting with different fruits and vegetables. Exchange recipes, tips, and success stories, fostering a supportive community around your juicing enthusiasm.

Finally, treat yourself to quality juicing equipment or accessories as a symbolic gesture of commitment to your well-being. Whether it's a stylish new juicer or vibrant glassware, these additions can elevate your juicing experience and serve as tangible reminders of your health-focused journey.

In essence, celebrating your juicing journey involves mindfulness, community, and self-care, turning a simple routine into a holistic celebration of vitality and good health.

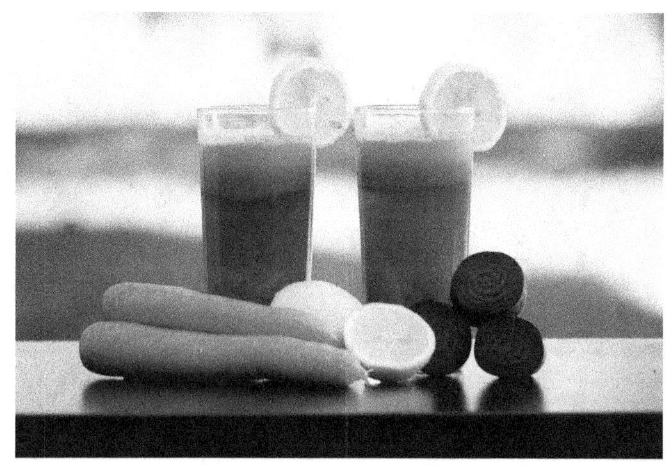

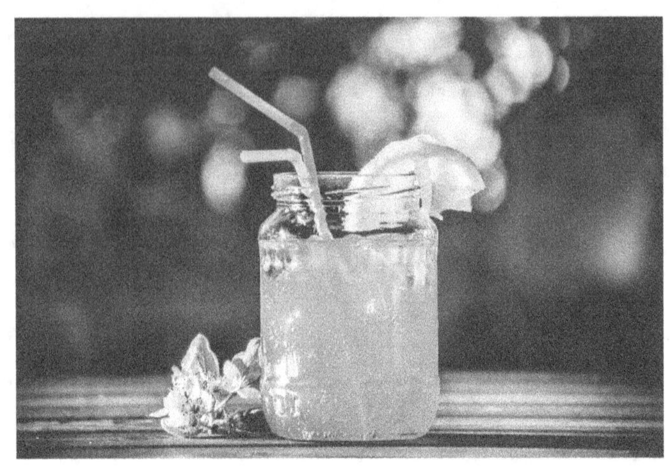

Conclusion

In conclusion, embarking on a juicing journey as a beginner can be a transformative and health-conscious choice. By incorporating fresh fruits and vegetables into a daily juicing routine, individuals can not only boost their nutrient intake but also enhance overall well-being. The ease of preparation, variety of flavor combinations, and potential health benefits make juicing an accessible and enjoyable lifestyle choice. However, it's essential to strike a balance, ensuring a diverse and balanced diet beyond just juices. With moderation and mindful choices, juicing can be a refreshing and delicious addition to a beginner's path towards a healthier lifestyle.

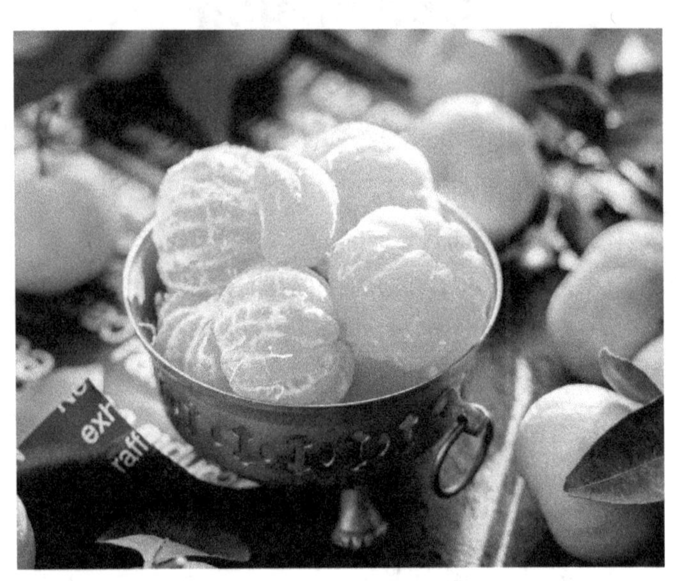